Just in Time for My

Just in Time for My

Karen L. Aken

ISBN-13: 978-1522990925

ISBN-10: 1522990925

Introduction

We all have something at some point in our lives that we want to look our best for, whether it be a wedding, high school reunion, or vacation. Why not use that excuse to get healthy once and for all? This guide gives you the tools to work towards getting in the best shape of your life now and beyond whatever special event you are preparing for. Write your reason for beginning this program on the cover. Inside you will find health tips and a direct guide for what you should be doing everyday or every other day (just remember to continue to drink your water, and eat your fruit and veggies on your off days). This program can take you as little as 3 months or as long as 6 months to complete, but my hope is that you will continue with these lifestyle changes for the rest of your life. Never go beyond your abilities. This guide is one of the simplest and most affordable ways to get healthy on your own.

The information in this book is not intended or implied to be a substitute for professional medical advice, diagnosis or treatment. All content contained in this book is for general information purposes only. Any reliance you place on such information is therefore strictly at your own risk.

Date:_____

Goal (daily or weekly):_____

Weight:_____

Cross the following items off this list once completed:

Walk for 5 minutes or jog for 3 minutes*

Do 10 Jumping Jacks

Stand on one leg for 10 seconds, then the other for 10 seconds

Do 10 arm circles forward, and 10 backwards

Suck in your stomach for 30 seconds

Drink 8 cups of water ** (Circle once completed) 1 2 3 4 5 6 7 8

Sit in silence for 5 minutes. Set a timer, silence your electronic devices, close your eyes, and take deep breaths until time is up.

Eat at least one piece of fruit.

Eat at least one half-cup serving of vegetables.

Choose at least one item from the following to eliminate from your diet:

Soda   Red Meat   Ice Cream   Potato Chips   Lunch Meat

*Decide now whether you want to walk or jog for this program, if you decide later to jog start with day one recommended amounts and work up. If you would like to push yourself even harder walk and jog the recommended amounts each day.

**JUST WATER, no added flavoring! Always drink clean, filtered water.

Date:_____

Goal:_____

Cross the following items off this list once completed:

Walk for 5 minutes or jog for 3 minutes

Do 10 Jumping Jacks

Stand on one leg for 10 seconds, then the other for 10 seconds*

Do 10 arm circles forward, and 10 backwards

Suck in your stomach for 30 seconds

Drink 8 cups of water 1 2 3 4 5 6 7 8

Sit in silence for 5 minutes. Set a timer, silence your electronic devices, close your eyes, and take deep breaths until time is up.

Eat at least one piece of fruit.

Eat at least one half-cup serving of vegetables.

Eliminated item(s)_____

*Standing on one leg improves your balance and also works your stomach muscles.

Date:_____

Goal:_____

Cross the following items off this list once completed:

Walk for 5 minutes or jog for 3 minutes

Do 10 Jumping Jacks

Stand on one leg for 10 seconds, then the other for 10 seconds

Do 10 arm circles forward, and 10 backwards

Suck in your stomach for 30 seconds

Drink 8 cups of water 1 2 3 4 5 6 7 8

Sit in silence for 5 minutes. Set a timer, silence your electronic devices, close your eyes, and take deep breaths until time is up.*

Eat at least one piece of fruit.

Eat at least one half-cup serving of vegetables.

Eliminated item(s)_____

*This exercise decreases cortisol, the hormone that contributes to increases in belly fat.

Date:_____

Goal:_____

Cross the following items off this list once completed:

Walk for 5 minutes or jog for 3 minutes

Do 10 Jumping Jacks

Stand on one leg for 10 seconds, then the other for 10 seconds

Do 10 arm circles forward, and 10 backwards

Suck in your stomach for 30 seconds

Drink 8 cups of water 1 2 3 4 5 6 7 8

Sit in silence for 5 minutes. Set a timer, silence your electronic devices, close your eyes, and take deep breaths until time is up.

Eat at least one piece of fruit.

Eat at least one half-cup serving of vegetables.*

Eliminated item(s)_____

*Fried vegetables have no nutritional value.

Date:_____

Goal:_____

Cross the following items off this list once completed:

Walk for 5 minutes or jog for 3 minutes

Do 10 Jumping Jacks

Stand on one leg for 10 seconds, then the other for 10 seconds

Do 10 arm circles forward, and 10 backwards

Suck in your stomach for 30 seconds

Drink 8 cups of water 1 2 3 4 5 6 7 8

Sit in silence for 5 minutes. Set a timer, silence your electronic devices, close your eyes, and take deep breaths until time is up.

Eat at least one piece of fruit.

Eat at least one half-cup serving of vegetables.

Eliminated item(s)_____

*Frozen fruits and vegetables are less expensive and contain more nutrients than canned.

Date:_____

Goal:_____

Cross the following items off this list once completed:

Walk for 5 minutes or jog for 3 minutes

Do 10 Jumping Jacks

Stand on one leg for 10 seconds, then the other for 10 seconds*

Do 10 arm circles forward, and 10 backwards

Suck in your stomach for 30 seconds

Drink 8 cups of water 1 2 3 4 5 6 7 8

Sit in silence for 5 minutes. Set a timer, silence your electronic devices, close your eyes, and take deep breaths until time is up.

Eat at least one piece of fruit.

Eat at least one half-cup serving of vegetables.

Eliminated item(s)_____

*Closing your eyes while standing on one leg makes every muscle used for balance in your body work even harder.

Date:_____

Goal:_____

Weight:_____

Cross the following items off this list once completed:

Walk for **10** minutes* or jog for **5** minutes

Do **15** Jumping Jacks

Stand on one leg for **15** seconds, then the other for **15** seconds

Do 10 arm circles forward, and 10 backwards

Suck in your stomach for 30 seconds

Look straight ahead, **kiss towards the sky 20x**

Drink 8 cups of water 1 2 3 4 5 6 7 8

Sit in silence for 5 minutes. Set a timer, silence your electronic devices, close your eyes, and take deep breaths until time is up.

Eat at least one piece of fruit.

Eat at least **one cup** of vegetables.

Eliminated item(s)_____

*If walking for 10 minutes is a bit strenuous then walk for 5 minutes in the morning and 5 in the afternoon.

Date:_____

Goal:_____

Cross the following items off this list once completed:

Walk for 10 minutes or jog for 5 minutes

Do 15 Jumping Jacks

Stand on one leg for 15 seconds, then the other for 15 seconds

Do 10 arm circles forward, and 10 backwards

Suck in your stomach for 30 seconds

Kiss toward the sky 20x*

Drink 8 cups of water 1 2 3 4 5 6 7 8

Sit in silence for 5 minutes. Set a timer, silence your electronic devices, close your eyes, and take deep breaths until time is up.

Eat at least one piece of fruit.

Eat at least one cup of vegetables.

Eliminated item(s)_____

*A little silly, but this exercise is one of the best ways to get rid of a double chin. If you're lucky enough to not have one it is still a great way to firm up that area.

Date:_____

Goal:_____

Cross the following items off this list once completed:

Walk for 10 minutes or jog for 5 minutes

Do 15 Jumping Jacks

Stand on one leg for 15 seconds, then the other for 15 seconds

Do 10 arm circles forward, and 10 backwards

Suck in your stomach for 30 seconds

Kiss toward the sky 20x

Drink 8 cups of water 1 2 3 4 5 6 7 8

Sit in silence for 5 minutes. Set a timer, silence your electronic devices, close your eyes, and take deep breaths until time is up.

Eat at least one piece of fruit.

Eat at least one cup of vegetables.

Eliminated item(s)_____

*Cut down on your to-do list. Write down your daily or weekly schedule, put them in order of important to least important, study the bottom of the list, is there anything you can remove from the list?

Date:_____

Goal:_____

Cross the following items off this list once completed:

Walk for 10 minutes or jog for 5 minutes

Do 15 Jumping Jacks

Stand on one leg for 15 seconds, then the other for 15 seconds

Do 10 arm circles forward, and 10 backwards

Suck in your stomach for 30 seconds

Kiss toward the sky 20x

Drink 8 cups of water 1 2 3 4 5 6 7 8

Sit in silence for 5 minutes. Set a timer, silence your electronic devices, close your eyes, and take deep breaths until time is up.

Eat at least one piece of fruit.

Eat at least one cup of vegetables.

Eliminated item(s)_____

*Get rid of your salt shaker and use Mrs. Dash to lower your sodium intake.

Date:_____

Goal:_____

Cross the following items off this list once completed:

Walk for 10 minutes or jog for 5 minutes

Do 15 Jumping Jacks

Stand on one leg for 15 seconds, then the other for 15 seconds

Do 10 arm circles forward, and 10 backwards

Suck in your stomach for 30 seconds

Kiss toward the sky 20x

Drink 8 cups of water 1 2 3 4 5 6 7 8

Sit in silence for 5 minutes. Set a timer, silence your electronic devices, close your eyes, and take deep breaths until time is up.

Eat at least one piece of fruit.

Eat at least one cup of vegetables.

Eliminated item(s)_____

*If you can't avoid eating something greasy, the least you can do is blot away the grease with a paper towel or napkin to slightly lower your fat intake.

Date:_____

Goal:_____

Cross the following items off this list once completed:

Walk for 10 minutes or jog for 5 minutes

Do 15 Jumping Jacks

Stand on one leg for 15 seconds, then the other for 15 seconds

Do 10 arm circles forward, and 10 backwards

Suck in your stomach for 30 seconds

Kiss toward the sky 20x

Drink 8 cups of water 1 2 3 4 5 6 7 8

Sit in silence for 5 minutes. Set a timer, silence your electronic devices, close your eyes, and take deep breaths until time is up.

Eat at least one piece of fruit.

Eat at least one cup of vegetables.

Eliminated item(s)_____

*When people eat slower they consume 10% less calories. Try taking smaller bites, chewing slowly, chewing until food in liquified or has lost texture, and finish chewing and swallowing completely before taking your next bite.

Date:_____

Goal:_____

Cross the following items off this list once completed:

Walk for 10 minutes or jog for 5 minutes

Do 15 Jumping Jacks

Stand on one leg for 15 seconds, then the other for 15 seconds

Do 10 arm circles forward, and 10 backwards

Suck in your stomach for 30 seconds

Kiss toward the sky 20x

Drink 8 cups of water 1 2 3 4 5 6 7 8

Sit in silence for 5 minutes. Set a timer, silence your electronic devices, close your eyes, and take deep breaths until time is up.

Eat at least one piece of fruit.

Eat at least one cup of vegetables.

Eliminated item(s)_____

*Drinking lots of water will not make you bloated. When you are well hydrated your body is less likely to hold onto excess fluids because it senses that is not at risk of dehydration.

Date:_____

Goal:_____

Weight:_____

Cross the following items off this list once completed:

Walk for **15** minutes or jog for **7** minutes

Do **20** Jumping Jacks

Stand on one leg for 15 seconds, then the other for 15 seconds

Do **15** arm circles forward, and **15** backwards

Suck in your stomach for 30 seconds, **wait 10 seconds, do it again**

Kiss toward the sky 20x

Drink 8 cups of water 1 2 3 4 5 6 7 8

Sit in silence for 5 minutes. Set a timer, silence your electronic devices, close your eyes, and take deep breaths until time is up.

Eat at least **two pieces** of fruit.

Eat at least one cup of vegetables.

Eliminated item(s)_____

Choose one, two, or all of the following groups of items from the following choices to eliminate from your diet*:

White Bread & Rice   Fried Foods   Cereal   Lunch Meat

*Replace white bread & rice with whole grain bread & rice, replace fried foods with baked, steamed, and/or boiled, replace cereal with gluten-free oatmeal, and replace lunch meat with peanut butter or lettuce, cucumber, and tomato with guacamole.

Date:_____

Goal:_____

Cross the following items off this list once completed:

Walk for 15 minutes or jog for 7 minutes

Do 20 Jumping Jacks

Stand on one leg for 15 seconds, then the other for 15 seconds

Do 15 arm circles forward, and 15 backwards

Suck in your stomach for 30 seconds, wait 10 seconds, do it again

Kiss toward the sky 20x

Drink 8 cups of water 1 2 3 4 5 6 7 8

Sit in silence for 5 minutes. Set a timer, silence your electronic devices, close your eyes, and take deep breaths until time is up.

Eat at least two pieces of fruit.

Eat at least one cup of vegetables.

Eliminated item(s)_____

*Microwave popcorn is not the healthy option people believe it to be, the chemicals found in microwave popcorn have been found to be carcinogenic.

Date:_____

Goal:_____

Cross the following items off this list once completed:

Walk for 15 minutes or jog for 7 minutes

Do 20 Jumping Jacks

Stand on one leg for 15 seconds, then the other for 15 seconds

Do 15 arm circles forward, and 15 backwards

Suck in your stomach for 30 seconds, wait 10 seconds, do it again

Kiss toward the sky 20x

Drink 8 cups of water 1 2 3 4 5 6 7 8

Sit in silence for 5 minutes. Set a timer, silence your electronic devices, close your eyes, and take deep breaths until time is up.

Eat at least two pieces of fruit.

Eat at least one cup of vegetables.

Eliminated item(s)_____

*If the first flour in the ingredient list is refined (ex. bleached or unbleached wheat flour) you are not getting 100% whole-grain.

Date:_____

Goal:_____

Cross the following items off this list once completed:

Walk for 15 minutes or jog for 7 minutes

Do 20 Jumping Jacks

Stand on one leg for 15 seconds, then the other for 15 seconds

Do 15 arm circles forward, and 15 backwards

Suck in your stomach for 30 seconds, wait 10 seconds, do it again

Kiss toward the sky 20x

Drink 8 cups of water 1 2 3 4 5 6 7 8

Sit in silence for 5 minutes. Set a timer, silence your electronic devices, close your eyes, and take deep breaths until time is up.

Eat at least two pieces of fruit.

Eat at least one cup of vegetables.

Eliminated item(s)_____

*The optimal room temperature for sleeping is 67 degrees.

Date:_____

Goal:_____

Cross the following items off this list once completed:

Walk for 15 minutes or jog for 7 minutes

Do 20 Jumping Jacks

Stand on one leg for 15 seconds, then the other for 15 seconds

Do 15 arm circles forward, and 15 backwards

Suck in your stomach for 30 seconds, wait 10 seconds, do it again

Kiss toward the sky 20x

Drink 8 cups of water 1 2 3 4 5 6 7 8

Sit in silence for 5 minutes. Set a timer, silence your electronic devices, close your eyes, and take deep breaths until time is up.

Eat at least two pieces of fruit.

Eat at least one cup of vegetables.

Eliminated item(s)_____

*Never go more than 4 hours without eating. Your body can jump into survival mode very quickly. Once in survival mode, your metabolism slows down.

Date:_____

Goal:_____

Cross the following items off this list once completed:

Walk for 15 minutes or jog for 7 minutes

Do 20 Jumping Jacks

Stand on one leg for 15 seconds, then the other for 15 seconds

Do 15 arm circles forward, and 15 backwards

Suck in your stomach for 30 seconds, wait 10 seconds, do it again

Kiss toward the sky 20x

Drink 8 cups of water 1 2 3 4 5 6 7 8

Sit in silence for 5 minutes. Set a timer, silence your electronic devices, close your eyes, and take deep breaths until time is up.

Eat at least two pieces of fruit.

Eat at least one cup of vegetables.

Eliminated item(s)_____

*Sit or stand while watching TV instead of lying down to burn more calories. Marching in place is even better.

Date:_____

Goal:_____

Cross the following items off this list once completed:

Walk for 15 minutes or jog for 7 minutes

Do 20 Jumping Jacks

Stand on one leg for 15 seconds, then the other for 15 seconds

Do 15 arm circles forward, and 15 backwards

Suck in your stomach for 30 seconds, wait 10 seconds, do it again

Kiss toward the sky 20x

Drink 8 cups of water 1 2 3 4 5 6 7 8

Sit in silence for 5 minutes. Set a timer, silence your electronic

devices, close your eyes, and take deep breaths until time is up.

Eat at least two pieces of fruit.

Eat at least one cup of vegetables.

Eliminated item(s)_____

*The high copper content found in peanut butter can prevent gray hair.

Date:_____

Goal:_____

Weight:_____

Cross the following items off this list once completed:

Walk for **20** minutes or jog for **9** minutes

Do 20 Jumping Jacks

Stand on one leg for **20** seconds, then the other for **20** seconds

Do 15 arm circles forward, and 15 backwards

Suck in your stomach for 30 seconds, wait 10 seconds, do it again

Your choice 10 sit-ups and/or pretend to hula-hoop in one direction for 30 seconds, then the other for 30 seconds

Kiss towards the sky **30x**

Drink **9** cups of water 1 2 3 4 5 6 7 8 9

Sit in silence for 5 minutes. Set a timer, silence your electronic devices, close your eyes, and take deep breaths until time is up.

Eat at least two pieces of fruit.

Eat at least **one and a half cups** of vegetables.

Eliminated item(s)_____

*People who fidget throughout the day can burn up to 350 more calories per day on average vs. people who sit still.

Date:_____

Goal:_____

Cross the following items off this list once completed:

Walk for 20 minutes or jog for 9 minutes

Do 20 Jumping Jacks

Stand on one leg for 20 seconds, then the other for 20 seconds

Do 15 arm circles forward, and 15 backwards

Suck in your stomach for 30 seconds, wait 10 seconds, do it again

Do 10 sit-ups and/or pretend to hula-hoop both directions for 30 seconds

Kiss towards the sky 30x

Drink 9 cups of water 1 2 3 4 5 6 7 8 9

Sit in silence for 5 minutes. Set a timer, silence your electronic devices, close your eyes, and take deep breaths until time is up.

Eat at least two pieces of fruit.

Eat at least one and a half cup serving of vegetables.

Eliminated item(s)_____

*Because broccoli is an excellent source of vitamin C it can help to shorten the duration of colds in the same way that oranges can.

Date:_____

Goal:_____

Cross the following items off this list once completed:

Walk for 20 minutes or jog for 9 minutes

Do 20 Jumping Jacks

Stand on one leg for 20 seconds, then the other for 20 seconds

Do 15 arm circles forward, and 15 backwards

Suck in your stomach for 30 seconds, wait 10 seconds, do it again

Do 10 sit-ups and/or pretend to hula-hoop both directions for 30 seconds

Kiss toward the sky 30x

Drink 9 cups of water 1 2 3 4 5 6 7 8 9

Sit in silence for 5 minutes. Set a timer, silence your electronic devices, close your eyes, and take deep breaths until time is up.

Eat at least two pieces of fruit.

Eat at least one and a half cup serving of vegetables.

Eliminated item(s)_____

*Walk like you are late. Use your arms more to pick up your speed (as mall walkers do). This can increase your calorie expenditure by up to 7%.

Date:_____

Goal:_____

Cross the following items off this list once completed:

Walk for 20 minutes or jog for 9 minutes

Do 20 Jumping Jacks

Stand on one leg for 20 seconds, then the other for 20 seconds

Do 15 arm circles forward, and 15 backwards

Suck in your stomach for 30 seconds, wait 10 seconds, do it again

Do 10 sit-ups and/or pretend to hula-hoop both directions for 30 seconds

Kiss toward the sky 30x

Drink 9 cups of water 1 2 3 4 5 6 7 8 9

Sit in silence for 5 minutes. Set a timer, silence your electronic devices, close your eyes, and take deep breaths until time is up.

Eat at least two pieces of fruit.

Eat at least one and a half cup serving of vegetables.

Eliminated item(s)_____

*Stand on your tippy toes while brushing your teeth to burn a few extra calories and improve your balance.

Date:_____

Goal:_____

Cross the following items off this list once completed:

Walk for 20 minutes or jog for 9 minutes

Do 20 Jumping Jacks

Stand on one leg for 20 seconds, then the other for 20 seconds

Do 15 arm circles forward, and 15 backwards

Suck in your stomach for 30 seconds, wait 10 seconds, do it again

Do 10 sit-ups and/or pretend to hula-hoop both directions for 30 seconds

Kiss toward the sky 30x

Drink 9 cups of water 1 2 3 4 5 6 7 8 9

Sit in silence for 5 minutes. Set a timer, silence your electronic devices, close your eyes, and take deep breaths until time is up.

Eat at least two pieces of fruit.

Eat at least one and a half cup serving of vegetables.

Eliminated item(s)_____

*Singing can burn 10-20 calories per song and improve your mood.

Date:_____

Goal:_____

Cross the following items off this list once completed:

Walk for 20 minutes or jog for 9 minutes

Do 20 Jumping Jacks

Stand on one leg for 20 seconds, then the other for 20 seconds

Do 15 arm circles forward, and 15 backwards

Suck in your stomach for 30 seconds, wait 10 seconds, do it again

Do 10 sit-ups and/or pretend to hula-hoop both directions for 30 seconds

Kiss toward the sky 30x

Drink 9 cups of water 1 2 3 4 5 6 7 8 9

Sit in silence for 5 minutes. Set a timer, silence your electronic devices, close your eyes, and take deep breaths until time is up.

Eat at least two pieces of fruit.

Eat at least one and a half cup serving of vegetables.

Eliminated item(s)_____

*Cut caffeine before 2 p.m. Caffeine can stay in your system for up to 8 hours and prevent you from falling asleep at night.

Date:_____

Goal:_____

Cross the following items off this list once completed:

Walk for 20 minutes or jog for 9 minutes

Do 20 Jumping Jacks

Stand on one leg for 20 seconds, then the other for 20 seconds

Do 15 arm circles forward, and 15 backwards

Suck in your stomach for 30 seconds, wait 10 seconds, do it again

Do 10 sit-ups and/or pretend to hula-hoop both directions for 30 seconds

Kiss toward the sky 30x

Drink 9 cups of water 1 2 3 4 5 6 7 8 9

Sit in silence for 5 minutes. Set a timer, silence your electronic devices, close your eyes, and take deep breaths until time is up.

Eat at least two pieces of fruit.

Eat at least one and a half cup serving of vegetables.

Eliminated item(s)_____

*If you would like to burn calories while waiting in line, march in place, do side leg raises, or alternate standing on one foot then the other, all while sucking in your stomach (just remember to breathe).

Date:_____

Goal:_____

Weight:_____

Cross the following items off this list once completed:

Walk for 20 minutes or jog for **11** minutes

Do **25** Jumping Jacks

Stand on one leg for 20 seconds, then the other for 20 seconds

Do **20** arm circles forward, and **20** backwards

Suck in your stomach for **45** seconds, wait 10 seconds, do it again

Do **15** sit-ups and/or pretend to hula-hoop both directions for **45** seconds

Kiss toward the sky 30x

Drink 9 cups of water 1 2 3 4 5 6 7 8 9

Sit in silence for 5 minutes. Set a timer, silence your electronic devices, close your eyes, and take deep breaths until time is up.

Eat at least two pieces of fruit.

Eat at least **two cups** of vegetables.

Eliminated item(s)_____

*Carbohydrates are good for you as long as you are choosing healthy carbs like whole grain bread, potatoes, fruits, and vegetables.

Date:_____

Goal:_____

Cross the following items off this list once completed:

Walk for 20 minutes or jog for 11 minutes

Do 25 Jumping Jacks

Stand on one leg for 20 seconds, then the other for 20 seconds

Do 20 arm circles forward, and 20 backwards

Suck in your stomach for 45 seconds, wait 10 seconds, do it again

Do 15 sit-ups and/or pretend to hula-hoop both directions for 45 seconds

Kiss toward the sky 30x

Drink 9 cups of water 1 2 3 4 5 6 7 8 9

Sit in silence for 5 minutes. Set a timer, silence your electronic devices, close your eyes, and take deep breaths until time is up.

Eat at least two pieces of fruit.

Eat at least two cups of vegetables.

Eliminated item(s)_____

*Carbohydrates should make up 45-65% of your caloric intake. Carbohydrates provide 4 calories per gram, to determine your recommended intake take 45-65% of your total daily caloric intake and then divide that number by 4.

Date:_____

Goal:_____

Cross the following items off this list once completed:

Walk for 20 minutes or jog for 11 minutes

Do 25 Jumping Jacks

Stand on one leg for 20 seconds, then the other for 20 seconds

Do 20 arm circles forward, and 20 backwards

Suck in your stomach for 45 seconds, wait 10 seconds, do it again

Do 15 sit-ups and/or pretend to hula-hoop both directions for 45 seconds

Kiss toward the sky 30x

Drink 9 cups of water 1 2 3 4 5 6 7 8 9

Sit in silence for 5 minutes. Set a timer, silence your electronic devices, close your eyes, and take deep breaths until time is up.

Eat at least two pieces of fruit.

Eat at least two cups of vegetables.

Eliminated item(s)_____

*You need some fat in your diet, just make sure you are consuming "healthy" fats like monounsaturated and polyunsaturated fats found in things like nuts, seeds, avocados, and olive oil.

Date:_____

Goal:_____

Cross the following items off this list once completed:

Walk for 20 minutes or jog for 11 minutes

Do 25 Jumping Jacks

Stand on one leg for 20 seconds, then the other for 20 seconds

Do 20 arm circles forward, and 20 backwards

Suck in your stomach for 45 seconds, wait 10 seconds, do it again

Do 15 sit-ups and/or pretend to hula-hoop both directions for 45 seconds

Kiss toward the sky 30x

Drink 9 cups of water 1 2 3 4 5 6 7 8 9

Sit in silence for 5 minutes. Set a timer, silence your electronic devices, close your eyes, and take deep breaths until time is up.

Eat at least two pieces of fruit.

Eat at least two cups of vegetables.

Eliminated item(s)_____

*Fat should make up 20-35% of your caloric intake. Fats provide 9 calories per gram, to determine your recommended intake take 20-35% of your total daily caloric intake and then divide that number by 9.

Date:_____

Goal:_____

Cross the following items off this list once completed:

Walk for 20 minutes or jog for 11 minutes

Do 25 Jumping Jacks

Stand on one leg for 20 seconds, then the other for 20 seconds

Do 20 arm circles forward, and 20 backwards

Suck in your stomach for 45 seconds, wait 10 seconds, do it again

Do 15 sit-ups and/or pretend to hula-hoop both directions for 45 seconds

Kiss toward the sky 30x

Drink 9 cups of water 1 2 3 4 5 6 7 8 9

Sit in silence for 5 minutes. Set a timer, silence your electronic devices, close your eyes, and take deep breaths until time is up.

Eat at least two pieces of fruit.

Eat at least two cups of vegetables.

Eliminated item(s)_____

*The more active you are the more protein you need. It is important that you consume enough protein to keep up with the body's constant breakdown and regeneration of the body's cells. Excess protein will be converted to fat because the body does not store protein for later use.

Date:_____

Goal:_____

Cross the following items off this list once completed:

Walk for 20 minutes or jog for 11 minutes

Do 25 Jumping Jacks

Stand on one leg for 20 seconds, then the other for 20 seconds

Do 20 arm circles forward, and 20 backwards

Suck in your stomach for 45 seconds, wait 10 seconds, do it again

Do 15 sit-ups and/or pretend to hula-hoop both directions for 45 seconds

Kiss toward the sky 30x

Drink 9 cups of water 1 2 3 4 5 6 7 8 9

Sit in silence for 5 minutes. Set a timer, silence your electronic devices, close your eyes, and take deep breaths until time is up.

Eat at least two pieces of fruit.

Eat at least two cups of vegetables.

Eliminated item(s)_____

*Protein should make up 15-35% of your caloric intake. Protein provides 4 calories per gram, to determine your recommended intake take 15-35% of your total daily caloric intake and then divide that number by 4. Intakes of 30-35% are only recommended for people who exercise for more than 60 minutes per day or who have a physically strenuous job.

Date:_____

Goal:_____

Cross the following items off this list once completed:

Walk for 20 minutes or jog for 11 minutes

Do 25 Jumping Jacks

Stand on one leg for 20 seconds, then the other for 20 seconds

Do 20 arm circles forward, and 20 backwards

Suck in your stomach for 45 seconds, wait 10 seconds, do it again

Do 15 sit-ups and/or pretend to hula-hoop both directions for 45 seconds

Kiss toward the sky 30x

Drink 9 cups of water 1 2 3 4 5 6 7 8 9

Sit in silence for 5 minutes. Set a timer, silence your electronic devices, close your eyes, and take deep breaths until time is up.

Eat at least two pieces of fruit.

Eat at least two cups of vegetables.

Eliminated item(s)_____

*The body needs sodium for normal heart rhythm, but only in moderation. Most people should aim to consume less than 2,400 mg of sodium per day. Consuming less than 1,500 mg can prevent and in some cases reverse heart disease. If you pay attention to nothing else you should at least pay attention to your sodium intake.

Date:_____

Goal:_____

Weight:_____

Cross the following items off this list once completed:

Walk for **25** minutes or jog for **13** minutes

Do 25 Jumping Jacks

Stand on one leg for **25** seconds, then the other for **25** seconds

Do 20 arm circles forward, and 20 backwards

Suck in your stomach for 45 seconds, wait 10 seconds, do it again

Do 15 sit-ups and/or pretend to hula-hoop both directions for 45 seconds

Chair squats. Stand in front of a couch or chair with your legs shoulder width apart, sit down just barely touching the chair and then stand back up again, repeat 5x*

Kiss toward the sky 30x

Drink 9 cups of water 1 2 3 4 5 6 7 8 9

Sit in silence for **7** minutes. Set a timer, silence your electronic devices, close your eyes, and take deep breaths until time is up.

Eat at least two pieces of fruit.

Eat at least **two and a half** cups of vegetables.

Eliminate something new (your choice)_____

Eliminated item(s)_____

*If at any time during this exercise you feel dizzy or out of breath please stop immediately. Do not attempt this exercise again, consult with your physician.

Date:_____

Goal:_____

Cross the following items off this list once completed:

Walk for 25 minutes or jog for 13 minutes

Do 25 Jumping Jacks

Stand on one leg for 25 seconds, then the other for 25 seconds

Do 20 arm circles forward, and 20 backwards

Suck in your stomach for 45 seconds, wait 10 seconds, do it again

Do 15 sit-ups and/or pretend to hula-hoop both directions for 45 seconds

Chair squats 5x*

Kiss toward the sky 30x

Drink 9 cups of water 1 2 3 4 5 6 7 8 9

Sit in silence for 7 minutes. Set a timer, silence your electronic devices, close your eyes, and take deep breaths until time is up.

Eat at least two pieces of fruit.

Eat at least two and a half cups of vegetables.

Eliminated item(s)_____

*This exercise is great for your hips, thighs, and backside.

Date:_____

Goal:_____

Cross the following items off this list once completed:

Walk for 25 minutes or jog for 13 minutes

Do 25 Jumping Jacks

Stand on one leg for 25 seconds, then the other for 25 seconds

Do 20 arm circles forward, and 20 backwards

Suck in your stomach for 45 seconds, wait 10 seconds, do it again

Do 15 sit-ups and/or pretend to hula-hoop both directions for 45 seconds

Chair squats 5x

Kiss toward the sky 30x

Drink 9 cups of water 1 2 3 4 5 6 7 8 9

Sit in silence for 7 minutes. Set a timer, silence your electronic devices, close your eyes, and take deep breaths until time is up.

Eat at least two pieces of fruit.

Eat at least two and a half cups of vegetables.

Eliminated item(s)_____

*Try using ground turkey instead of ground beef. Though the fat content may be the same, ground beef will have more saturated fat.

Date:_____

Goal:_____

Cross the following items off this list once completed:

Walk for 25 minutes or jog for 13 minutes

Do 25 Jumping Jacks

Stand on one leg for 25 seconds, then the other for 25 seconds

Do 20 arm circles forward, and 20 backwards

Suck in your stomach for 45 seconds, wait 10 seconds, do it again

Do 15 sit-ups and/or pretend to hula-hoop both directions for 45 seconds

Chair squats 5x

Kiss toward the sky 30x

Drink 9 cups of water 1 2 3 4 5 6 7 8 9

Sit in silence for 7 minutes. Set a timer, silence your electronic devices, close your eyes, and take deep breaths until time is up.

Eat at least two pieces of fruit.

Eat at least two and a half cups of vegetables.

Eliminated item(s)_____

*Breathing from your abdomen instead of your chest can improve your health in many ways. To see what type of breather you are, lay down, place one hand on your chest and one on your abdomen. If the hand on your chest rises more, you are a chest breather, if the hand on your abdomen rises more you are an abdomen breather.

Date:_____

Goal:_____

Cross the following items off this list once completed:

Walk for 25 minutes or jog for 13 minutes

Do 25 Jumping Jacks

Stand on one leg for 25 seconds, then the other for 25 seconds

Do 20 arm circles forward, and 20 backwards

Suck in your stomach for 45 seconds, wait 10 seconds, do it again

Do 15 sit-ups and/or pretend to hula-hoop both directions for 45 seconds

Chair squats 5x

Kiss toward the sky 30x

Drink 9 cups of water 1 2 3 4 5 6 7 8 9

Sit in silence for 7 minutes. Set a timer, silence your electronic devices, close your eyes, and take deep breaths until time is up.

Eat at least two pieces of fruit.

Eat at least two and a half cups of vegetables.

Eliminated item(s)_____

*To practice abdominal breathing, sit comfortably. Rest your hand lightly on your abdomen (about an inch from your navel) so that you can get a better sense of it's movement. Inhale slowly for 4 seconds, pause for 2 seconds, then exhale for 4 seconds. Repeat for as long or as little as you like.

Date:_____

Goal:_____

Cross the following items off this list once completed:

Walk for 25 minutes or jog for 13 minutes

Do 25 Jumping Jacks

Stand on one leg for 25 seconds, then the other for 25 seconds

Do 20 arm circles forward, and 20 backwards

Suck in your stomach for 45 seconds, wait 10 seconds, do it again

Do 15 sit-ups and/or pretend to hula-hoop both directions for 45 seconds

Chair squats 5x

Kiss toward the sky 30x

Drink 9 cups of water 1 2 3 4 5 6 7 8 9

Sit in silence for 7 minutes. Set a timer, silence your electronic devices, close your eyes, and take deep breaths until time is up.

Eat at least two pieces of fruit.

Eat at least two and a half cups of vegetables.

Eliminated item(s)_____

*Stair climbing is classified as a "vigorous" exercise and burns more calories per minute than jogging.

Date:_____

Goal:_____

Cross the following items off this list once completed:

Walk for 25 minutes or jog for 13 minutes

Do 25 Jumping Jacks

Stand on one leg for 25 seconds, then the other for 25 seconds

Do 20 arm circles forward, and 20 backwards

Suck in your stomach for 45 seconds, wait 10 seconds, do it again

Do 15 sit-ups and/or pretend to hula-hoop both directions for 45 seconds

Chair squats 5x

Kiss toward the sky 30x

Drink 9 cups of water 1 2 3 4 5 6 7 8 9

Sit in silence for 7 minutes. Set a timer, silence your electronic devices, close your eyes, and take deep breaths until time is up.

Eat at least two pieces of fruit.

Eat at least two and a half cups of vegetables.

Eliminated item(s)_____

*Try switching your salad dressing to salsa to cut back on calories, fat, and sugar, but be wary of the amount of sodium salsa may have.

Date:_____

Goal:_____

Weight:_____

Cross the following items off this list once completed:

Walk for 25 minutes or jog for 15 minutes

Do **30** Jumping Jacks

Stand on one leg for 25 seconds, then the other for 25 seconds

Do 20 arm circles forward, and 20 backwards

Suck in your stomach for **60** seconds, wait 10 seconds, do it again

Do 20 sit-ups and/or pretend to hula-hoop both directions for **60** seconds

Chair squats **7x**

Kiss toward the sky **35x**

Drink 9 cups of water 1 2 3 4 5 6 7 8 9

Sit in silence for 7 minutes. Set a timer, silence your electronic devices, close your eyes, and take deep breaths until time is up.

Eat at least **three** pieces of fruit.

Eat at least two and a half cups of vegetables.

Eliminated item(s)_____

*Orange fruits and vegetables are good for your eyes, skin, and immunity.

Date:_____

Goal:_____

Cross the following items off this list once completed:

Walk for 25 minutes or jog for 15 minutes

Do 30 Jumping Jacks

Stand on one leg for 25 seconds, then the other for 25 seconds

Do 20 arm circles forward, and 20 backwards

Suck in your stomach for 60 seconds, wait 10 seconds, do it again

Do 20 sit-ups and/or pretend to hula-hoop both directions for 60 seconds

Chair squats 7x

Kiss toward the sky 35x

Drink 9 cups of water 1 2 3 4 5 6 7 8 9

Sit in silence for 7 minutes. Set a timer, silence your electronic devices, close your eyes, and take deep breaths until time is up.

Eat at least three pieces of fruit.

Eat at least two and a half cups of vegetables.

Eliminated item(s)_____

*Green fruits and vegetables are good for your eyes, bones, and teeth.

Date:_____

Goal:_____

Cross the following items off this list once completed:

Walk for 25 minutes or jog for 15 minutes

Do 30 Jumping Jacks

Stand on one leg for 25 seconds, then the other for 25 seconds

Do 20 arm circles forward, and 20 backwards

Suck in your stomach for 60 seconds, wait 10 seconds, do it again

Do 20 sit-ups and/or pretend to hula-hoop both directions for 60 seconds

Chair squats 7x

Kiss toward the sky 35x

Drink 9 cups of water 1 2 3 4 5 6 7 8 9

Sit in silence for 7 minutes. Set a timer, silence your electronic devices, close your eyes, and take deep breaths until time is up.

Eat at least three pieces of fruit.

Eat at least two and a half cups of vegetables.

Eliminated item(s)_____

*Yellow fruits and vegetables are good for your skin, teeth, and bones.

Date:_____

Goal:_____

Cross the following items off this list once completed:

Walk for 25 minutes or jog for 15 minutes

Do 30 Jumping Jacks

Stand on one leg for 25 seconds, then the other for 25 seconds

Do 20 arm circles forward, and 20 backwards

Suck in your stomach for 60 seconds, wait 10 seconds, do it again

Do 20 sit-ups and/or pretend to hula-hoop both directions for 60 seconds

Chair squats 7x

Kiss toward the sky 35x

Drink 9 cups of water 1 2 3 4 5 6 7 8 9

Sit in silence for 7 minutes. Set a timer, silence your electronic devices, close your eyes, and take deep breaths until time is up.

Eat at least three pieces of fruit.

Eat at least two and a half cups of vegetables.

Eliminated item(s)_____

*Purple fruits and vegetables are good for your heart and liver.

Date:_____

Goal:_____

Cross the following items off this list once completed:

Walk for 25 minutes or jog for 15 minutes

Do 30 Jumping Jacks

Stand on one leg for 25 seconds, then the other for 25 seconds

Do 20 arm circles forward, and 20 backwards

Suck in your stomach for 60 seconds, wait 10 seconds, do it again

Do 20 sit-ups and/or pretend to hula-hoop both directions for 60 seconds

Chair squats 7x

Kiss toward the sky 35x

Drink 9 cups of water 1 2 3 4 5 6 7 8 9

Sit in silence for 7 minutes. Set a timer, silence your electronic devices, close your eyes, and take deep breaths until time is up.

Eat at least three pieces of fruit.

Eat at least two and a half cups of vegetables.

Eliminated item(s)_____

*White fruits and vegetables are good for your bones.

Date:_____

Goal:_____

Cross the following items off this list once completed:

Walk for 25 minutes or jog for 15 minutes

Do 30 Jumping Jacks

Stand on one leg for 25 seconds, then the other for 25 seconds

Do 20 arm circles forward, and 20 backwards

Suck in your stomach for 60 seconds, wait 10 seconds, do it again

Do 20 sit-ups and/or pretend to hula-hoop both directions for 60 seconds

Chair squats 7x

Kiss toward the sky 35x

Drink 9 cups of water 1 2 3 4 5 6 7 8 9

Sit in silence for 7 minutes. Set a timer, silence your electronic devices, close your eyes, and take deep breaths until time is up.

Eat at least three pieces of fruit.

Eat at least two and a half cups of vegetables.

Eliminated item(s)_____

*Red fruits and vegetables are good for your heart.

Date:_____

Goal:_____

Cross the following items off this list once completed:

Walk for 25 minutes or jog for 15 minutes

Do 30 Jumping Jacks

Stand on one leg for 25 seconds, then the other for 25 seconds

Do 20 arm circles forward, and 20 backwards

Suck in your stomach for 60 seconds, wait 10 seconds, do it again

Do 20 sit-ups and/or pretend to hula-hoop both directions for 60 seconds

Chair squats 7x

Kiss toward the sky 35x

Drink 9 cups of water 1 2 3 4 5 6 7 8 9

Sit in silence for 7 minutes. Set a timer, silence your electronic devices, close your eyes, and take deep breaths until time is up.

Eat at least three pieces of fruit.

Eat at least two and a half cups of vegetables.

Eliminated item(s)_____

*Gatorade and other sports drinks are just as unhealthy for you as soda because of their high salt and sugar content. They are only appropriate for vigorous intensity exercisers and those who live or work in hot climates.

Date:_____

Goal:_____

Weight:_____

Cross the following items off this list once completed:

Walk for **30** minutes or jog for **17** minutes

Do 30 Jumping Jacks

Stand on one leg for **30** seconds, then the other for **30** seconds

Do **25** arm circles forward, and **25** backwards

Suck in your stomach for 60 seconds, wait 10 seconds, do it again

Do 20 sit-ups and/or pretend to hula-hoop both directions for 60 seconds

Chair squats **9x**

Kiss toward the sky 35x

Drink 9 cups of water 1 2 3 4 5 6 7 8 9

Sit in silence for 7 minutes. Set a timer, silence your electronic devices, close your eyes, and take deep breaths until time is up.

Eat at least three pieces of fruit.

Eat at least two and a half cups of vegetables.

Eliminated item(s)_____

*Try to avoid purchasing canned food. Canned food contains high amounts of sodium and preservatives that can wreak havoc on your body. If you must purchase canned foods such as beans or vegetables, dump them in a strainer and rinse them with water to eliminate most of the sodium.

Date:_____

Goal:_____

Cross the following items off this list once completed:

Walk for 30 minutes or jog for 17 minutes

Do 30 Jumping Jacks

Stand on one leg for 30 seconds, then the other for 30 seconds

Do 25 arm circles forward, and 25 backwards

Suck in your stomach for 60 seconds, wait 10 seconds, do it again

Do 20 sit-ups and/or pretend to hula-hoop both directions for 60 seconds

Chair squats 9x

Kiss toward the sky 35x

Drink 9 cups of water 1 2 3 4 5 6 7 8 9

Sit in silence for 7 minutes. Set a timer, silence your electronic devices, close your eyes, and take deep breaths until time is up.

Eat at least three pieces of fruit.

Eat at least two and a half cups of vegetables.

Eliminated item(s)_____

*Avoid high fructose corn syrup as often as possible. It has been linked to many diseases including type 2 diabetes and fibromyalgia. Most generic products have high fructose corn syrup because it is a cheap alternative to real sugar.

Date:_____

Goal:_____

Cross the following items off this list once completed:

Walk for 30 minutes or jog for 17 minutes

Do 30 Jumping Jacks

Stand on one leg for 30 seconds, then the other for 30 seconds

Do 25 arm circles forward, and 25 backwards

Suck in your stomach for 60 seconds, wait 10 seconds, do it again

Do 20 sit-ups and/or pretend to hula-hoop both directions for 60 seconds

Chair squats 9x

Kiss toward the sky 35x

Drink 9 cups of water 1 2 3 4 5 6 7 8 9

Sit in silence for 7 minutes. Set a timer, silence your electronic devices, close your eyes, and take deep breaths until time is up.

Eat at least three pieces of fruit.

Eat at least two and a half cups of vegetables.

Eliminated item(s)_____

*Artificial light can make it harder for your body to recognize when it is time to sleep. If you have a hard time falling asleep at night make sure you stop using electronic devices at least 30 minutes before bed, make your bedroom as dark as possible, and face any alarm clocks away from your eyes.

Date:_____

Goal:_____

Cross the following items off this list once completed:

Walk for 30 minutes or jog for 17 minutes

Do 30 Jumping Jacks

Stand on one leg for 30 seconds, then the other for 30 seconds

Do 25 arm circles forward, and 25 backwards

Suck in your stomach for 60 seconds, wait 10 seconds, do it again

Do 20 sit-ups and/or pretend to hula-hoop both directions for 60 seconds

Chair squats 9x

Kiss toward the sky 35x

Drink 9 cups of water 1 2 3 4 5 6 7 8 9

Sit in silence for 7 minutes. Set a timer, silence your electronic devices, close your eyes, and take deep breaths until time is up.

Eat at least three pieces of fruit.

Eat at least two and a half cups of vegetables.

Eliminated item(s)_____

*Certain foods burn more calories than others. This is called the thermic effect of food or TEF. Examples of foods with a higher TEF are: egg whites, chicken, turkey, salmon, oatmeal, yams, multi-grain cereals, and whole grain bread.

Date:_____

Goal:_____

Cross the following items off this list once completed:

Walk for 30 minutes or jog for 17 minutes

Do 30 Jumping Jacks

Stand on one leg for 30 seconds, then the other for 30 seconds

Do 25 arm circles forward, and 25 backwards

Suck in your stomach for 60 seconds, wait 10 seconds, do it again

Do 20 sit-ups and/or pretend to hula-hoop both directions for 60 seconds

Chair squats 9x

Kiss toward the sky 35x

Drink 9 cups of water 1 2 3 4 5 6 7 8 9

Sit in silence for 7 minutes. Set a timer, silence your electronic devices, close your eyes, and take deep breaths until time is up.

Eat at least three pieces of fruit.

Eat at least two and a half cups of vegetables.

Eliminated item(s)_____

*Lunch meats are processed with nitrates that are carcinogenic. They also contain high amounts of sodium and sugar. Lunch meat has been linked to stomach cancer, colon cancer, and type 2 diabetes.

Date:_____

Goal:_____

Cross the following items off this list once completed:

Walk for 30 minutes or jog for 17 minutes

Do 30 Jumping Jacks

Stand on one leg for 30 seconds, then the other for 30 seconds

Do 25 arm circles forward, and 25 backwards

Suck in your stomach for 60 seconds, wait 10 seconds, do it again

Do 20 sit-ups and/or pretend to hula-hoop both directions for 60 seconds

Chair squats 9x

Kiss toward the sky 35x

Drink 9 cups of water 1 2 3 4 5 6 7 8 9

Sit in silence for 7 minutes. Set a timer, silence your electronic devices, close your eyes, and take deep breaths until time is up.

Eat at least three pieces of fruit.

Eat at least two and a half cups of vegetables.

Eliminated item(s)_____

*Cutting calories below 1200 is dangerous and should only be done when under the supervision of a physician.

Date:_____

Goal:_____

Cross the following items off this list once completed:

Walk for 30 minutes or jog for 17 minutes

Do 30 Jumping Jacks

Stand on one leg for 30 seconds, then the other for 30 seconds

Do 25 arm circles forward, and 25 backwards

Suck in your stomach for 60 seconds, wait 10 seconds, do it again

Do 20 sit-ups and/or pretend to hula-hoop both directions for 60 seconds

Chair squats 9x

Kiss toward the sky 35x

Drink 9 cups of water 1 2 3 4 5 6 7 8 9

Sit in silence for 7 minutes. Set a timer, silence your electronic devices, close your eyes, and take deep breaths until time is up.

Eat at least three pieces of fruit.

Eat at least two and a half cups of vegetables.

Eliminated item(s)_____

*If you do not have a lot of time, exercising in bouts of at least 10 minutes at a time is still beneficial.

Date:_____

Goal:_____

Weight:_____

Cross the following items off this list once completed:

Walk for 30 minutes or jog for **19** minutes

Do 30 Jumping Jacks

Stand on one leg for 30 seconds, then the other for 30 seconds

Do 25 arm circles forward, and 25 backwards

Suck in your stomach for 60 seconds, wait 10 seconds, **repeat 2x**

Do **25** sit-ups and/or pretend to hula-hoop both directions for **75** seconds

Chair squats **10x**

Kiss toward the sky 35x

Drink 9 cups of water 1 2 3 4 5 6 7 8 9

Sit in silence for 7 minutes. Set a timer, silence your electronic devices, close your eyes, and take deep breaths until time is up.

Eat at least three pieces of fruit.

Eat at least two and a half cups of vegetables.

Eliminate something new (your choice)_____

Eliminated item(s)_____

*A healthy diet is not one that is low in fat, carbs, and calories. A healthy diet is nutrient dense. When you fulfill your body's nutritional needs it can run more efficiently.

Date:_____

Goal:_____

Cross the following items off this list once completed:

Walk for 30 minutes or jog for 19 minutes

Do 30 Jumping Jacks

Stand on one leg for 30 seconds, then the other for 30 seconds

Do 25 arm circles forward, and 25 backwards

Suck in your stomach for 60 seconds, wait 10 seconds, repeat 2x

Do 25 sit-ups and/or pretend to hula-hoop both directions for 75 seconds

Chair squats 10x

Kiss toward the sky 35x

Drink 9 cups of water 1 2 3 4 5 6 7 8 9

Sit in silence for 7 minutes. Set a timer, silence your electronic devices, close your eyes, and take deep breaths until time is up.

Eat at least three pieces of fruit.

Eat at least two and a half cups of vegetables.

Eliminated item(s)_____

*Always leave time for laughing. Laughing is good for your mind, body, and soul.

Date:_____

Goal:_____

Cross the following items off this list once completed:

Walk for 30 minutes or jog for 19 minutes

Do 30 Jumping Jacks

Stand on one leg for 30 seconds, then the other for 30 seconds

Do 25 arm circles forward, and 25 backwards

Suck in your stomach for 60 seconds, wait 10 seconds, repeat 2x

Do 25 sit-ups and/or pretend to hula-hoop both directions for 75 seconds

Chair squats 10x

Kiss toward the sky 35x

Drink 9 cups of water 1 2 3 4 5 6 7 8 9

Sit in silence for 7 minutes. Set a timer, silence your electronic devices, close your eyes, and take deep breaths until time is up.

Eat at least three pieces of fruit.

Eat at least two and a half cups of vegetables.

Eliminated item(s)_____

*Going to bed at the same time every day and waking up at the same time every day will set your internal body clock. This will make it easier to fall asleep, wake up, and leave you feeling less tired in the morning.

Date:_____

Goal:_____

Cross the following items off this list once completed:

Walk for 30 minutes or jog for 19 minutes

Do 30 Jumping Jacks

Stand on one leg for 30 seconds, then the other for 30 seconds

Do 25 arm circles forward, and 25 backwards

Suck in your stomach for 60 seconds, wait 10 seconds, repeat 2x

Do 25 sit-ups and/or pretend to hula-hoop both directions for 75 seconds

Chair squats 10x

Kiss toward the sky 35x

Drink 9 cups of water 1 2 3 4 5 6 7 8 9

Sit in silence for 7 minutes. Set a timer, silence your electronic devices, close your eyes, and take deep breaths until time is up.

Eat at least three pieces of fruit.

Eat at least two and a half cups of vegetables.

Eliminated item(s)_____

*Avoid people who stress you out. If someone consistently causes emotional stress in your life avoid them completely or limit the amount of time you spend with them.

Date:_____

Goal:_____

Cross the following items off this list once completed:

Walk for 30 minutes or jog for 19 minutes

Do 30 Jumping Jacks

Stand on one leg for 30 seconds, then the other for 30 seconds

Do 25 arm circles forward, and 25 backwards

Suck in your stomach for 60 seconds, wait 10 seconds, repeat 2x

Do 25 sit-ups and/or pretend to hula-hoop both directions for 75 seconds

Chair squats 10x

Kiss toward the sky 35x

Drink 9 cups of water 1 2 3 4 5 6 7 8 9

Sit in silence for 7 minutes. Set a timer, silence your electronic devices, close your eyes, and take deep breaths until time is up.

Eat at least three pieces of fruit.

Eat at least two and a half cups of vegetables.

Eliminated item(s)_____

*Breakfast should be eaten within 2 hours of waking up to keep your metabolism up, and also to give your mind and body energy.

Date:_____

Goal:_____

Cross the following items off this list once completed:

Walk for 30 minutes or jog for 19 minutes

Do 30 Jumping Jacks

Stand on one leg for 30 seconds, then the other for 30 seconds

Do 25 arm circles forward, and 25 backwards

Suck in your stomach for 60 seconds, wait 10 seconds, repeat 2x

Do 25 sit-ups and/or pretend to hula-hoop both directions for 75 seconds

Chair squats 10x

Kiss toward the sky 35x

Drink 9 cups of water 1 2 3 4 5 6 7 8 9

Sit in silence for 7 minutes. Set a timer, silence your electronic devices, close your eyes, and take deep breaths until time is up.

Eat at least three pieces of fruit.

Eat at least two and a half cups of vegetables.

Eliminated item(s)_____

*Swinging on a swing burns 100 calories in 30 minutes.

Date:_____

Goal:_____

Cross the following items off this list once completed:

Walk for 30 minutes or jog for 19 minutes

Do 30 Jumping Jacks

Stand on one leg for 30 seconds, then the other for 30 seconds

Do 25 arm circles forward, and 25 backwards

Suck in your stomach for 60 seconds, wait 10 seconds, repeat 2x

Do 25 sit-ups and/or pretend to hula-hoop both directions for 75 seconds

Chair squats 10x

Kiss toward the sky 35x

Drink 9 cups of water 1 2 3 4 5 6 7 8 9

Sit in silence for 7 minutes. Set a timer, silence your electronic devices, close your eyes, and take deep breaths until time is up.

Eat at least three pieces of fruit.

Eat at least two and a half cups of vegetables.

Eliminated item(s)_____

*Listening to music improves memory and mood.

Date:_____

Goal:_____

Weight:_____

Cross the following items off this list once completed:

Walk for **35** minutes or jog for **21** minutes

Do **35** Jumping Jacks

Stand on one leg for **35** seconds, then the other for **35** seconds

Do **30** arm circles forward, and **30** backwards

Suck in your stomach for 60 seconds, wait 10 seconds, repeat 2x

Do 25 sit-ups and/or pretend to hula-hoop both directions for 75 seconds

Chair squats 10x

Kiss toward the sky 35x

Drink 9 cups of water 1 2 3 4 5 6 7 8 9

Sit in silence for 7 minutes. Set a timer, silence your electronic devices, close your eyes, and take deep breaths until time is up.

Eat at least three pieces of fruit.

Eat at least two and a half cups of vegetables.

Eliminated item(s)_____

*Cinnamon lowers blood sugar, increases metabolism, and helps fight against bacterial and fungal infections. Avoid supplements, instead try to add cinnamon whenever possible to foods that could use a bit of extra flavor.

Date:_____

Goal:_____

Cross the following items off this list once completed:

Walk for 35 minutes or jog for 21 minutes

Do 35 Jumping Jacks

Stand on one leg for 35 seconds, then the other for 35 seconds

Do 30 arm circles forward, and 30 backwards

Suck in your stomach for 60 seconds, wait 10 seconds, repeat 2x

Do 25 sit-ups and/or pretend to hula-hoop both directions for 75 seconds

Chair squats 10x

Kiss toward the sky 35x

Drink 9 cups of water 1 2 3 4 5 6 7 8 9

Sit in silence for 7 minutes. Set a timer, silence your electronic devices, close your eyes, and take deep breaths until time is up.

Eat at least three pieces of fruit.

Eat at least two and a half cups of vegetables.

Eliminated item(s)_____

*Berries are one of the best sources of antioxidants. They aid in weight loss because of their high water and fiber content.

Date:_____

Goal:_____

Cross the following items off this list once completed:

Walk for 35 minutes or jog for 21 minutes

Do 35 Jumping Jacks

Stand on one leg for 35 seconds, then the other for 35 seconds

Do 30 arm circles forward, and 30 backwards

Suck in your stomach for 60 seconds, wait 10 seconds, repeat 2x

Do 25 sit-ups and/or pretend to hula-hoop both directions for 75 seconds

Chair squats 10x

Kiss toward the sky 35x

Drink 9 cups of water 1 2 3 4 5 6 7 8 9

Sit in silence for 7 minutes. Set a timer, silence your electronic devices, close your eyes, and take deep breaths until time is up.

Eat at least three pieces of fruit.

Eat at least two and a half cups of vegetables.

Eliminated item(s)_____

*Honey can ease nighttime coughing. Never give honey to infants less than 12 months old.

Date:_____

Goal:_____

Cross the following items off this list once completed:

Walk for 35 minutes or jog for 21 minutes

Do 35 Jumping Jacks

Stand on one leg for 35 seconds, then the other for 35 seconds

Do 30 arm circles forward, and 30 backwards

Suck in your stomach for 60 seconds, wait 10 seconds, repeat 2x

Do 25 sit-ups and/or pretend to hula-hoop both directions for 75 seconds

Chair squats 10x

Kiss toward the sky 35x

Drink 9 cups of water 1 2 3 4 5 6 7 8 9

Sit in silence for 7 minutes. Set a timer, silence your electronic devices, close your eyes, and take deep breaths until time is up.

Eat at least three pieces of fruit.

Eat at least two and a half cups of vegetables.

Eliminated item(s)_____

*Cherries can help reduce arthritic inflammation.

Date:_____

Goal:_____

Cross the following items off this list once completed:

Walk for 35 minutes or jog for 21 minutes

Do 35 Jumping Jacks

Stand on one leg for 35 seconds, then the other for 35 seconds

Do 30 arm circles forward, and 30 backwards

Suck in your stomach for 60 seconds, wait 10 seconds, repeat 2x

Do 25 sit-ups and/or pretend to hula-hoop both directions for 75 seconds

Chair squats 10x

Kiss toward the sky 35x

Drink 9 cups of water 1 2 3 4 5 6 7 8 9

Sit in silence for 7 minutes. Set a timer, silence your electronic devices, close your eyes, and take deep breaths until time is up.

Eat at least three pieces of fruit.

Eat at least two and a half cups of vegetables.

Eliminated item(s)_____

*Peanut butter contains healthy fats and is rich in protein. Low fat peanut butters typically contain more chemicals, sugar, and salt to make up for the loss of flavor when fat is taken out.

Date:_____

Goal:_____

Cross the following items off this list once completed:

Walk for 35 minutes or jog for 21 minutes

Do 35 Jumping Jacks

Stand on one leg for 35 seconds, then the other for 35 seconds

Do 30 arm circles forward, and 30 backwards

Suck in your stomach for 60 seconds, wait 10 seconds, repeat 2x

Do 25 sit-ups and/or pretend to hula-hoop both directions for 75 seconds

Chair squats 10x

Kiss toward the sky 35x

Drink 9 cups of water 1 2 3 4 5 6 7 8 9

Sit in silence for 7 minutes. Set a timer, silence your electronic devices, close your eyes, and take deep breaths until time is up.

Eat at least three pieces of fruit.

Eat at least two and a half cups of vegetables.

Eliminated item(s)_____

*One bowl of oatmeal (preferably gluten free) per day can lower cholesterol and stabilize blood sugar.

Date:_____

Goal:_____

Cross the following items off this list once completed:

Walk for 35 minutes or jog for 21 minutes

Do 35 Jumping Jacks

Stand on one leg for 35 seconds, then the other for 35 seconds

Do 30 arm circles forward, and 30 backwards

Suck in your stomach for 60 seconds, wait 10 seconds, repeat 2x

Do 25 sit-ups and/or pretend to hula-hoop both directions for 75 seconds

Chair squats 10x

Kiss toward the sky 35x

Drink 9 cups of water 1 2 3 4 5 6 7 8 9

Sit in silence for 7 minutes. Set a timer, silence your electronic devices, close your eyes, and take deep breaths until time is up.

Eat at least three pieces of fruit.

Eat at least two and a half cups of vegetables.

Eliminated item(s)_____

*For a power breakfast try my Super Oatmeal:

1/4 - 1/2 cup gluten free quick oats, 1/2 - 3/4 cup water, Frozen Berries (your preferred amount and type), 1 3/4 tbs of peanut butter or 1 small spoonful of honey or agave, and 1/2 tsp cinnamon. Combine oats, water, berries, cinnamon in a bowl, cook for 1-2 min, stir in peanut butter or honey/agave.

Date:_____

Goal:_____

Weight:_____

Cross the following items off this list once completed:

Walk for **40** minutes or jog for **23** minutes

Do 35 Jumping Jacks

Stand on one leg for 35 seconds, then the other for 35 seconds

Do **35** arm circles forward, and **35** backwards

Suck in your stomach for 60 seconds, wait 10 seconds, **repeat 3x**

Do **30** sit-ups and/or pretend to hula-hoop both directions for **90** seconds

Chair squats **12x**

Kiss toward the sky **40x**

Drink 9 cups of water 1 2 3 4 5 6 7 8 9

Sit in silence for 7 minutes. Set a timer, silence your electronic devices, close your eyes, and take deep breaths until time is up.

Eat at least three pieces of fruit.

Eat at least two and a half cups of vegetables.

Eliminated item(s)_____

*Try to have at least 3 servings of whole grains per day. Look for the yellow whole grain stamp to ensure you truly are getting whole grains.

Date:_____

Goal:_____

Cross the following items off this list once completed:

Walk for 40 minutes or jog for 23 minutes

Do 35 Jumping Jacks

Stand on one leg for 35 seconds, then the other for 35 seconds

Do 35 arm circles forward, and 35 backwards

Suck in your stomach for 60 seconds, wait 10 seconds, repeat 3x

Do 30 sit-ups and/or pretend to hula-hoop both directions for 90 seconds

Chair squats 12x

Kiss toward the sky 40x

Drink 9 cups of water 1 2 3 4 5 6 7 8 9

Sit in silence for 7 minutes. Set a timer, silence your electronic devices, close your eyes, and take deep breaths until time is up.

Eat at least three pieces of fruit.

Eat at least two and a half cups of vegetables.

Eliminated item(s)_____

*When eating out, choose salmon over steak for heart healthy fats.

Date:_____

Goal:_____

Cross the following items off this list once completed:

Walk for 40 minutes or jog for 23 minutes

Do 35 Jumping Jacks

Stand on one leg for 35 seconds, then the other for 35 seconds

Do 35 arm circles forward, and 35 backwards

Suck in your stomach for 60 seconds, wait 10 seconds, repeat 3x

Do 30 sit-ups and/or pretend to hula-hoop both directions for 90 seconds

Chair squats 12x

Kiss toward the sky 40x

Drink 9 cups of water 1 2 3 4 5 6 7 8 9

Sit in silence for 7 minutes. Set a timer, silence your electronic devices, close your eyes, and take deep breaths until time is up.

Eat at least three pieces of fruit.

Eat at least two and a half cups of vegetables.

Eliminated item(s)_____

*The quercetin found in onions makes them a natural antihistamine (as long as they have not been battered and fried).

Date:_____

Goal:_____

Cross the following items off this list once completed:

Walk for 40 minutes or jog for 23 minutes

Do 35 Jumping Jacks

Stand on one leg for 35 seconds, then the other for 35 seconds

Do 35 arm circles forward, and 35 backwards

Suck in your stomach for 60 seconds, wait 10 seconds, repeat 3x

Do 30 sit-ups and/or pretend to hula-hoop both directions for 90 seconds

Chair squats 12x

Kiss toward the sky 40x

Drink 9 cups of water 1 2 3 4 5 6 7 8 9

Sit in silence for 7 minutes. Set a timer, silence your electronic devices, close your eyes, and take deep breaths until time is up.

Eat at least three pieces of fruit.

Eat at least two and a half cups of vegetables.

Eliminated item(s)_____

*Bell peppers are a good source of fiber, vitamin c, and antioxidants.

Date:_____

Goal:_____

Cross the following items off this list once completed:

Walk for 40 minutes or jog for 23 minutes

Do 35 Jumping Jacks

Stand on one leg for 35 seconds, then the other for 35 seconds

Do 35 arm circles forward, and 35 backwards

Suck in your stomach for 60 seconds, wait 10 seconds, repeat 3x

Do 30 sit-ups and/or pretend to hula-hoop both directions for 90 seconds

Chair squats 12x

Kiss toward the sky 40x

Drink 9 cups of water 1 2 3 4 5 6 7 8 9

Sit in silence for 7 minutes. Set a timer, silence your electronic devices, close your eyes, and take deep breaths until time is up.

Eat at least three pieces of fruit.

Eat at least two and a half cups of vegetables.

Eliminated item(s)_____

*Mushrooms are a good source of iron and help lower cholesterol.

Date:_____

Goal:_____

Cross the following items off this list once completed:

Walk for 40 minutes or jog for 23 minutes

Do 35 Jumping Jacks

Stand on one leg for 35 seconds, then the other for 35 seconds

Do 35 arm circles forward, and 35 backwards

Suck in your stomach for 60 seconds, wait 10 seconds, repeat 3x

Do 30 sit-ups and/or pretend to hula-hoop both directions for 90 seconds

Chair squats 12x

Kiss toward the sky 40x

Drink 9 cups of water 1 2 3 4 5 6 7 8 9

Sit in silence for 7 minutes. Set a timer, silence your electronic devices, close your eyes, and take deep breaths until time is up.

Eat at least three pieces of fruit.

Eat at least two and a half cups of vegetables.

Eliminated item(s)_____

*You can still eat the foods you love, just find simple ways to make recipes healthier, try lower fat cheeses, use herbs and spices instead of salt, or add extra vegetables such as carrots, broccoli, onions, green beens or peas to every dish. Try meatless spaghetti with chopped zucchini; experiment with spaghetti squash; or try bean and cheese tacos with shredded carrots, and diced onions instead of beef tacos (use vegetarian refried beans to avoid animal fats).

Date:_____

Goal:_____

Cross the following items off this list once completed:

Walk for 40 minutes or jog for 23 minutes

Do 35 Jumping Jacks

Stand on one leg for 35 seconds, then the other for 35 seconds

Do 35 arm circles forward, and 35 backwards

Suck in your stomach for 60 seconds, wait 10 seconds, repeat 3x

Do 30 sit-ups and/or pretend to hula-hoop both directions for 90 seconds

Chair squats 12x

Kiss toward the sky 40x

Drink 9 cups of water 1 2 3 4 5 6 7 8 9

Sit in silence for 7 minutes. Set a timer, silence your electronic devices, close your eyes, and take deep breaths until time is up.

Eat at least three pieces of fruit.

Eat at least two and a half cups of vegetables.

Eliminated item(s)_____

*Want pizza but not the fat and calories? Try thin crust pizza burgers:

2 packages of Oroweat Multigrain Sandwich Thins or Equivalent

Organic Pizza Sauce (Muir Glen or Dei Fratelli)

1 package shredded mozzarella cheese

Toppings: nothing canned, try a bag of frozen peppers, onions, spinach, and/or mushrooms. Bake for 20 minutes at 400 degrees, because ovens vary check pizza burgers at 15 minutes.

Date:_____

Goal:_____

Weight:_____

Cross the following items off this list once completed:

Walk for **45** minutes or jog for **25** minutes

Do **40** Jumping Jacks

Stand on one leg for **40** seconds, then the other for **40** seconds

Do **40** arm circles forward, and **40** backwards

Suck in your stomach for 60 seconds, wait 10 seconds, **repeat 4x**

Do **35** sit-ups and/or pretend to hula-hoop both directions for 2 minutes

Chair squats **15x**

Kiss toward the sky 40x

Drink 9 cups of water 1 2 3 4 5 6 7 8 9

Sit in silence for **10** minutes. Set a timer, silence your electronic devices, close your eyes, and take deep breaths until time is up.

Eat at least three pieces of fruit.

Eat at least two and a half cups of vegetables.

Eliminate something new (your choice)_____

Eliminated item(s)_____

*If you have met your goal create a new one or update the old one.

Date:_____

Goal:_____

Cross the following items off this list once completed:

Walk for 45 minutes or jog for 25 minutes

Do 40 Jumping Jacks

Stand on one leg for 40 seconds, then the other for 40 seconds

Do 40 arm circles forward, and 40 backwards

Suck in your stomach for 60 seconds, wait 10 seconds, repeat 4x

Do 35 sit-ups and/or pretend to hula-hoop both directions for 2 minutes

Chair squats 15x

Kiss toward the sky 40x

Drink 9 cups of water 1 2 3 4 5 6 7 8 9

Sit in silence for 10 minutes. Set a timer, silence your electronic devices, close your eyes, and take deep breaths until time is up.

Eat at least three pieces of fruit.

Eat at least two and a half cups of vegetables.

Eliminated item(s)_____

*Just 5-15 minutes of sunlight on your hands, arms, and face 2-3x each week can improve vitamin D production, reduce depression, and strengthen your bones.

Date:_____

Goal:_____

Cross the following items off this list once completed:

Walk for 45 minutes or jog for 25 minutes

Do 40 Jumping Jacks

Stand on one leg for 40 seconds, then the other for 40 seconds

Do 40 arm circles forward, and 40 backwards

Suck in your stomach for 60 seconds, wait 10 seconds, repeat 4x

Do 35 sit-ups and/or pretend to hula-hoop both directions for 2 minutes

Chair squats 15x

Kiss toward the sky 40x

Drink 9 cups of water 1 2 3 4 5 6 7 8 9

Sit in silence for 10 minutes. Set a timer, silence your electronic devices, close your eyes, and take deep breaths until time is up.

Eat at least three pieces of fruit.

Eat at least two and a half cups of vegetables.

Eliminated item(s)_____

*For a change of pace, pick out a fun workout video that involves weights, alternate between walking or jogging and the video.

Date:_____

Goal:_____

Cross the following items off this list once completed:

Walk for 45 minutes or jog for 25 minutes

Do 40 Jumping Jacks

Stand on one leg for 40 seconds, then the other for 40 seconds

Do 40 arm circles forward, and 40 backwards

Suck in your stomach for 60 seconds, wait 10 seconds, repeat 4x

Do 35 sit-ups and/or pretend to hula-hoop both directions for 2 minutes

Chair squats 15x

Kiss toward the sky 40x

Drink 9 cups of water 1 2 3 4 5 6 7 8 9

Sit in silence for 10 minutes. Set a timer, silence your electronic devices, close your eyes, and take deep breaths until time is up.

Eat at least three pieces of fruit.

Eat at least two and a half cups of vegetables.

Eliminated item(s)_____

*If your mind wanders at night keep a notebook by your bed and write down your thoughts. This is one of the easiest ways to get the thoughts out of your head. Tell yourself you will deal with them in the morning.

Date:_____

Goal:_____

Cross the following items off this list once completed:

Walk for 45 minutes or jog for 25 minutes

Do 40 Jumping Jacks

Stand on one leg for 40 seconds, then the other for 40 seconds

Do 40 arm circles forward, and 40 backwards

Suck in your stomach for 60 seconds, wait 10 seconds, repeat 4x

Do 35 sit-ups and/or pretend to hula-hoop both directions for 2 minutes

Chair squats 15x

Kiss toward the sky 40x

Drink 9 cups of water 1 2 3 4 5 6 7 8 9

Sit in silence for 10 minutes. Set a timer, silence your electronic devices, close your eyes, and take deep breaths until time is up.

Eat at least three pieces of fruit.

Eat at least two and a half cups of vegetables.

Eliminated item(s)_____

*In times of stress, inhale deeply for 5 seconds, pause for 3 seconds, and then exhale for 5 seconds. Repeat as necessary. This is one of the quickest ways to relax your body and lower your blood pressure.

Date:_____

Goal:_____

Cross the following items off this list once completed:

Walk for 45 minutes or jog for 25 minutes

Do 40 Jumping Jacks

Stand on one leg for 40 seconds, then the other for 40 seconds

Do 40 arm circles forward, and 40 backwards

Suck in your stomach for 60 seconds, wait 10 seconds, repeat 4x

Do 35 sit-ups and/or pretend to hula-hoop both directions for 2 minutes

Chair squats 15x

Kiss toward the sky 40x

Drink 9 cups of water 1 2 3 4 5 6 7 8 9

Sit in silence for 10 minutes. Set a timer, silence your electronic devices, close your eyes, and take deep breaths until time is up.

Eat at least three pieces of fruit.

Eat at least two and a half cups of vegetables.

Eliminated item(s)_____

*Learn how to say "no". Whether in your personal or professional life taking on more than you can handle only leads to stress. Your heart and mind will thank you.

Date:_____

Goal:_____

Cross the following items off this list once completed:

Walk for 45 minutes or jog for 25 minutes

Do 40 Jumping Jacks

Stand on one leg for 40 seconds, then the other for 40 seconds

Do 40 arm circles forward, and 40 backwards

Suck in your stomach for 60 seconds, wait 10 seconds, repeat 4x

Do 35 sit-ups and/or pretend to hula-hoop both directions for 2 minutes

Chair squats 15x

Kiss toward the sky 40x

Drink 9 cups of water 1 2 3 4 5 6 7 8 9

Sit in silence for 10 minutes. Set a timer, silence your electronic devices, close your eyes, and take deep breaths until time is up.

Eat at least three pieces of fruit.

Eat at least two and a half cups of vegetables.

Eliminated item(s)_____

*For a healthy salad that won't leave you feeling hungry, try making a Rainbow Salad:

1 to 2 cups red cabbage (cut or ripped into bite size pieces)

1 pouch 100 calorie guacamole (found in refrigerated veggie section) or 3 tbs. vegetarian refried beans

1/4 - 1/2 cup shredded carrots

1-2 tbs. salsa

To retain the health benefits you have achieved please continue with this program indefinitely. Your goal should be to complete the list 5-7x per week. Feel free to lengthen the time you walk or run to a time that is appropriate for you. You can also choose to do more of any of the other exercises on the list or keep the number of repetitions the same.

Cross the following items off this list once completed:
Walk for 45 minutes or jog for 25 minutes
Do 40 Jumping Jacks
Stand on one leg for 40 seconds, then the other for 40 seconds
Do 40 arm circles forward, and 40 backwards
Suck in your stomach for 60 seconds, wait 10 seconds, repeat 4x
Do 35 sit-ups and/or pretend to hula-hoop both directions for 2 minutes
Chair squats 15x
Kiss toward the sky 40x
Drink 9 cups of water 1 2 3 4 5 6 7 8 9
Sit in silence for 10 minutes. Set a timer, silence your electronic devices, close your eyes, and take deep breaths until time is up.
Eat at least three pieces of fruit.
Eat at least two and a half cups of vegetables.
Eliminated item(s)_____

Walk for 45 minutes or jog for 25 minutes

Do 40 Jumping Jacks

Stand on one leg for 40 seconds, then the other for 40 seconds

Do 40 arm circles forward, and 40 backwards

Suck in your stomach for 60 seconds, wait 10 seconds, repeat 4x

Do 35 sit-ups and/or pretend to hula-hoop both directions for 2 minutes

Chair squats 15x

Kiss toward the sky 40x

Drink 9 cups of water 1 2 3 4 5 6 7 8 9

Sit in silence for 10 minutes. Set a timer, silence your electronic devices, close your eyes, and take deep breaths until time is up.

Eat at least three pieces of fruit.

Eat at least two and a half cups of vegetables.

Eliminated item(s)_____

Walk for __ minutes or jog for__ minutes

Do __ Jumping Jacks

Stand on one leg for __ seconds, then the other for __ seconds

Do __ arm circles forward, and __ backwards

Suck in your stomach for __ seconds, wait __ seconds, repeat __x

Do __ sit-ups and/or pretend to hula-hoop both directions for __ minutes

Chair squats __x

Kiss toward the sky __x

Drink 9 cups of water 1 2 3 4 5 6 7 8 9

Sit in silence for __ minutes. Set a timer, silence your electronic devices, close your eyes, and take deep breaths until time is up.

Eat at least three pieces of fruit.

Eat at least two and a half cups of vegetables.

Eliminated item(s)_____

www.ingramcontent.com/pod-product-compliance
Lightning Source LLC
Chambersburg PA
CBHW050506290526
45786CB00006B/2455